I0408288

YOGA: THE UNIVERSAL GUIDE

CELEBRATING YOGA FOR THE BODY, MIND AND SOUL

BY DOMINIQUE ATKINSON

© 2017 by Dominique Atkinson
© 2017 by ALEX-PUBLISHING

All rights reserved

Published by:

ALEX-PUBLISHING

© Copyright 2017

All rights reserved. No part of this book may be reproduced or transmitted in any form or by any means, electronically or mechanically, including photocopy, recording, or by and information storage or retrieval system, without the written permission from the publisher, except in the case of brief quotations embodied in critical articles or reviews.

Trademarks are the property of their respective holders. When used, trademarks are for the benefit of the trademark owner only.

DISCLAIMER

The information provided herein is stated to be truthful and consistent, in that any liability, in terms of inattention or otherwise, by any usage or abusage of any policies, processes, or directions contained within is the solitary and utter responsibility of the recipient reader. Under no circumstances will any legal responsibility or blame be held against the publisher for any reparation, damages, or monetary loss due to the information herein, either directly or indirectly. Respective authors hold all rights not held by publisher.

Authors Note

Welcome to the amazing world of Yoga! As many of you know from my other books, this has been a passion of mine for more than 20 years. I'm blessed to have had incredible teacher's that have guided me in my practice, and I'm thrilled that you will allow me to help you learn the art of yoga. From whatever place you approach Yoga, you will surely find yourself with greater health, a calmer mind and a more peaceful spirit.

When reading through this book, remember that there is no right or wrong way to do yoga. The success is in the practice, not the outcome. Having said that, if you find that a certain yoga practice does not seem to be doing much for you, feel free to choose another one until you find your path to enlightenment and inner peace!

Yoga is a practice that everyone is familiar with in this modern age. Not everyone knows what it is, or why people choose to do it, but it is definitely not a foreign concept to most. What many people do not understand, however, is that there is so much more to yoga than an exercise regime. Of course it is one of the most effective ways to lose weight, lose stress, and gain confidence, but did you know that it is an excellent way to also gain control of your mind? There is so much more to yoga than what meets the eye. It isn't an exercise that people do, it is a lifestyle that people live.

Join me on this journey of discovering yoga. In this book, we are going to explore what yoga is, where it came from, and what it's all about. It doesn't matter if you are a beginner, or a seasoned Namaste enthusiast, this book has a lot to offer you. You aren't going to merely learn about yoga… you are going to learn how to experience yoga. We are going to look at how it affects every part of life, from losing weight and stress to gaining wisdom and confidence. This is a journey that welcomes all, no matter where you are in your life.

If you are already one that enjoys yoga, then you know that there is never a time in your life when you have achieved. There is always going to be room for improvement, and there is always going to be something to learn.

Yoga is not for the impatient one, and it is not for the person that wants to get things immediately. What yoga is, and who it is for are people who want to take control of their lives and know that there is a subtle healing in everything that they do. This is not an exercise regime, this is a lifestyle that will take you a lifetime to master and flourish in.

Best,

Dominique Atkinson

Table of Contents

What is Yoga? An Overview

Close your eyes for a second, and clear your mind. Once you have a clear mind, think of the word *yoga,* and focus on what comes to mind. For many people this is simple. Calm settings, mats, trendy pants and things of the sort. This isn't wrong by any means, these are all things that are associated with yoga, but these are not what yoga is about. There is so much more to the practice than what comes to mind when you think of the word.

This lifestyle originated in the country of India tens of thousands of years ago. It was first observed by the monks that had the understanding that this is a beneficial lifestyle to live, not only for yourself, but also for the rest of the world.

One who practices yoga as it was meant to be practiced is one that knows what it is like to need, and to share with others. They are a person that can recognize when someone else is in need of something, and they seek to help them.

This is not a selfish way to be, but rather a life that feeds off of the positivity of others, and the world surrounding us. When you embrace this practice for what it really is, you will find that you are gaining wisdom, confidence, and kindness as the days go by, without having to do a lot to your own mindset.

This is because that emotional response to this is involuntary. Yoga feeds off of the energy that is in the world. The more positive the energy, the better it is for everyone.

Yoga is not something that is practiced for a few hours a day a few times a week. Sure, that is a way to gain flexibility and maybe lose a few pounds, but there is so much more to it. You are missing out on so much if that is how you partake in yoga, and we strongly encourage you to reconsider how you are doing this, and what you can do to make it better.

Within days of doing yoga the right way... actually living it... you will find that you are calmer, easier going, and more relaxed. It will be as though someone has just lifted a major burden off of your shoulders, and has thrown it far away, never to be worried about again.

No matter where you are in your life, or what you need to accomplish yet, you can start practicing this life changing art at any time. Don't let anyone tell you that you don't have time, or the money, or that you need to be at a certain fitness level before you are able to partake.

This is a practice for everyone, and the more you get to live it, the better you will feel, and the better off the world will be. Come, embark on this journey, and discover the world you have been looking for.

The Building Blocks

"The journey of a thousand miles begins with the first step." These great words by the revered teacher Lao Tzu still ring true to this day. When you are setting out to do anything, whether it be something small that you will accomplish in one day, or something that is going to last you the rest of your life, you need to begin with the first step.

As with everything else on this planet, yoga is a practice that needs to be built off of the blocks from which it is composed. This means that you need to be ready to start on this journey, and you need to have a few things in order to do that.

Of course equipment is always optional, your own body weight and the comfort of your own home is enough to effectively practice yoga without a lot of problems, but there is a lot of benefits that do come from having the right tools for the trade.

Yoga mats are not essential, but you will be thrilled if you have one

Likely the most basic, yet also one of the biggest pieces of yoga equipment that you will ever use is the yoga m3at. We call it big in the sense that it is important, for it is far from a big piece of equipment.

Why are they so important? That's easy. They provide a surface for you to grip when you are in different positions. They provide a clean area for you to lay, especially if you are working out in a studio, and they help visualize where you should be placing your feet and hands.

That last one is especially important for those that are just starting out in this field. You will notice that your instructor will often tell you to put your feet at the base of your mat, or place your hands on either side of your mat.

Another common one is to keep your feet mat width apart. Of course you can do all of these things without a mat. They are really just spacing and placement of where you need to put things, but you will find that it is a lot easier to accomplish if you have a mat as a guide.

Yoga pants may be common place out on the street, but they really were meant for yoga.

Yoga pants are something that you can see virtually anywhere now. People where them for a variety of purposes, including as just regular pants these days, but their main purpose really was for yoga.

Yoga pants are form fitting, they are breathable, and they stretch. These are all things that make them perfect for this practice. It doesn't matter what shape you are bent in to, your pants will stay with you and never ride up or down.

For the workout, these really are a miracle, and if you do not already have some, you should definitely look into getting a pair. What makes them even better? The fact they come in all different kinds of colors and styles, so you can be yourself and get your workout in all at the same time.

Yoga socks... often overlooked, but they really are worth it.

Socks with no toes seem to be almost pointless, then throw in the fact that yoga socks don't have heels either, and you have a perfectly good reason to question why people wear them at all.

The answer is support. Yoga is a regime that requires you to move in so many different ways. Sure, they are natural, but not at first, and until your body is used to it, you are going to have to take it slow to keep from hurting yourself.

The arch and ankle support that yoga socks provide really is worth the cost and effort of getting a pair. More and more people are seeing this, so the socks are becoming more readily available, but if you still can't find a pair in your store then you should definitely look online.

There aren't any toes or heels so you can still grip your mat no matter what position you are in, yet there is a noticeable amount of support there so you don't have to worry about rolling your foot the wrong way or causing strain on your arch.

Shirts and wristbands may be the final touches to an outfit, but they are not any less important than the other things.

Wrist bands provide a lot of support for you in all of your new movements. You won't always need to use them, and you will actually find that your wrists do feel better even after your workout is completed, but in the meantime make sure you are wearing them for your workouts.

If you are wearing a shirt specifically to get the most out of your yoga regime, make sure the shirt you purchase is breathable, but that it also provides support. You don't want to have to worry about ripping or tearing anything when you are bending over or twisting around. The main purpose of all of the stretching is to relieve stress, so don't cause yourself more stress by wondering if you are going to tear your shirt during your workout.

As we said before, you don't need to have any of these things to have a successful yoga workout, and you especially don't need them for your yoga lifestyle, but you do need to realize that they will help you a lot with what you are doing.

There is no shame in being prepared, and there is nothing cool about a person that is putting themselves at risk by not doing something right out of fear of looking foolish.

Don't be the fool and try to show off. A wise person never feels the need to show off, and they always know that they need to do what is best for them and for those who are around them. Take the time to get at least the basic equipment before you start.

You will be really glad that you did.

Common Positions

So many people use the excuse that they don't like to work out in public, or that they don't have the money for yoga class. Yes, these may be valid points for someone who doesn't want to be exposed when they are working out, but they are not valid points to avoid doing yoga.

The most common of all yoga positions are easy to learn, and easy to practice. They won't cost you a dime to do them, and you don't ever have to do a single position in front of another person if you don't want to, although you will find that the more you do them, the more comfortable you will feel doing them and the more likely you will be to do them in front of others.

Before we get into all of those different positions, however, we are going to look at how you should breathe. Yoga breathing is different than regular breathing, and you need to make a deliberate effort to learn how to do it.

For starters, take a deep breath in, but open the back of your throat as you do it and breathe in through your nose. Take a deep breathe, not a shallow one, and not a regular one, but one that is actually cleansing.

You want to breathe in all of the positive, and breathe out the negative, and to do that you need to take in those long, deep breaths and force out all of that bad air through your mouth.

Practice breathing this way for a few minutes, when you have it down, you are ready to begin. Don't get discouraged if it takes you a while to get it, this is a lot harder to do then it sounds, but don't worry, anyone can do it, and everyone learns how to eventually.

Cross legged seated position
One of the most basic positions, all you have to do to do this pose is sit cross legged with your wrists on your knees, palms turned upward. Keep your eyes closed and just breathe.

Table top position
This position requires you to be on your hands and knees, with your knees straight out behind you, and the tops of your feet pressed against the floor. Keep your back flat, your tummy pulled firmly in, and your neck straight.

You will be looking down at the floor as you do this position, and just breathe. You will feel this in your abs and arms, and the cleansing will be good for your soul.

Cat pose
Start in the table top pose, then, when you are ready, arch your back and breathe in. Lower your back as far as you can without bending your arms or legs, and breathe out. Repeat this as many times as you would like.

It creates flexibility in your spine, and helps to align everything in your core. If you feel nauseous doing this pose, try slowing it down. There is no rush in any of yoga, let everything you do be slow and deliberate, as one who is on a mission.

Cobra pose

Start by lying flat on your face with your arms down by your side. When you are ready, bring your hands up and place them by your head, then lift yourself up off of the floor, only leaving your legs on the floor entirely.

Press the tops of your feet into the floor, and arch your back. Look up to the sky and breathe in and out, enjoying the stretch in your back and neck.

Downward dog pose

Begin lying on your face just as you did with the cobra pose. This time, raise your butt off of the mat and push your hands down into the floor. Press your feet firmly on the floor as well, and hold this pose.

You should look as though you are forming a triangle with your body, pressing your hands and feet firmly against the floor as you keep your tummy pulled in and your tail bone down.

Breathe in and out, and relax.

Child's pose

Sit on your legs with your legs bent as though you were doing something on your lap. When you are ready, lean forward, only bending at the torso, and stretch your arms out as far in front of you as you can.

Place your hands on the floor, and press your palms into the floor. Keep your eyes closed and your face downward, and breathe. This is a perfect pose to meditate in, and you can hold it comfortably for hours.

Stretching out the bottom of your back and the top of your thighs, you will find that this is a great pose for flexibility.

All of these poses are great for those who have never before done yoga, and they are also a great pose to return to if you are a seasoned enthusiast. There is never a point when you outgrow a pose, no matter how long you have been doing yoga.

To make any of these poses more difficult, try sinking down deeper into them, or try raising a foot or a hand. See how long you can hold a pose that requires you to use more of your internal muscles and less of your balance.

There is always a way to make these poses a little bit harder if you would like to, and you will always benefit from working at it. Don't ever give up on a pose because you find it difficult. Life throws challenges our way to make us grow, not to make us shrink away from what we are to do.

If you view every opportunity or problem that comes your way as a growing experience, you will find that your circumstances sky rocket. This is not because they will get easier, or that they will change, but that you will change.

There is so much good that having a good attitude can do for you, and all you have to do is try. Next time you are faced with a challenge, take it head on and throw all you have into the opportunity.

Attitude affects a lot of what we do, and when you have a good attitude, there is nothing that can stand in your way.

Losing Weight with Yoga

There are hundreds of different kinds of people that partake in yoga, and their reasons for doing so are as varied as they are. One of the top three reasons that people start practicing yoga, however, is for the weight loss benefits.

There are a lot of people out there who have lost a lot of weight using yoga alone. They never had to run on a treadmill, they never had to do sit ups, pull ups, or crunches, in fact, they didn't have to do anything vigorous or rigorous.

Sound too good to be true? Well, it's not. If you want to practice yoga simply because you are wanting to lose some weight, you are in luck. Yoga works out every part of the body, deep inside where there are little muscles that no one thinks about, to carving those sexy abs that we all wish we had.

What determines how much you will lose with yoga is how much you are putting into the practice. Yoga itself burns plenty of calories, but there are different workouts you can do that will help you burn off those calories better.

If you look virtually anywhere, you will find that there are different kinds of yoga workouts based on your own specific preference or need. If you want to still have the different days that you work on different parts of your body, go for it.

There are yoga poses that specifically target different parts of your body, and there are also yoga regimes that target your entire body for entire body weight loss.

One of the major benefits of losing weight with yoga is that you can track with results within the first week. It is a workout that requires a lot of flexibility, and even if you are not a flexible person when you begin, you will see a drastic improvement by the end of week 1.

When you are a month in, you will see even more. There really is no end to how fast you see improvements in your body when you are using yoga for weight loss. Another added benefit of yoga versus other forms of exercise is that yoga will tone as you go.

You don't just lose the weight and become skinny, you lose the weight and become a lean, toned, flexible machine. And what you gain is so much more than just a new body. You will find that you are more relaxed, that your health is better, and that you have a better lookout on life when you are practicing yoga.

To gain a better understanding as to why this is so effective, let's take a look at what it is yoga actually does when you are working out. There is the ever popular high intensity interval training when it comes to working out, and this seems like the opposite of that, but it is just as effective, so why is that?

Let's take a look at the core. Literally. When you are doing a yoga pose, you are often required to hold that pose for a length of time, often a minute or two. That sounds easy enough, but when you are actually doing it, you will find that you feel shaky, and like your muscles are weak.

This is because yoga works deep inside with muscles, all of those little muscles that we often ignore as we are seeking a six pack. What makes yoga so effective is that you don't have to try to target these muscles, it just happens from the position you are in.

And if you add to that the fact you have to fight to keep your balance during many of the poses, you will find that the amount of calories that your body burns while doing a pose sky rockets as opposed to doing the same thing with both of your feet planted firmly on the floor.

You may think that you need to do a lot of jumping around to get your heart rate up, after all, isn't that what Richard Simmons taught us back in the day? While it is true you need to get your heart rate up to burn off extra calories and strengthen your heart, it isn't true that you need to do a lot of aerobics to get it up.

If you do a regime in yoga, and go through a variety of poses without stopping and repeat the same set over for a couple of times, odds are you won't be able to keep up at first.

There is a lot more to this exercising than what meets the eye, and you will be amazed at how much is really required of you when you are doing a workout. It isn't a bad thing, in fact, this is really good. You don't have to worry that you will injure yourself going at some crazy move, but you will still get great, fat burning benefits, just like you would if you were doing a lot of jumping jacks, or some other exercise they said you had to do to be fit.

As with any weight loss goal, you need to set healthy standards and follow through with them, but we promise you that if you work hard at it, and stay consistent, you will find that your weight loss goals are easy to achieve, and you don't have to do anything but incorporate yoga into your day.

Eating Well Living Well

Those who actively enjoy participating in yoga for a lifestyle have reported that they prefer to eat better when they are practicing. This has a lot of different benefits that are all wonderful, but it really helps in the matter of weight loss.

A lot of people mistakenly think that if they want to lose weight, that means they have to deprive themselves and not ever have anything that they like. This is far from true, and I will tell you why.

Calories are in food. They are in everything that we put into our bodies, whether it be a vegetable or a piece of candy, to everything in between. What the game is when you are trying to lose weight, is to eat (we have to eat, starvation is never an option, besides who doesn't like to eat, anyway?), but not to overdo the calories.

Truth be told, the foods that many of us prefer, processed foods, candy, desserts, sodas, and things that are along those lines, are filled with what is known as empty calories.

That means you are eating, you are not getting full, or if you are full you will find that you are hungry again within a short period of time, and you are eating way more calories than the energy that is provided.

When food enters our bodies, or body uses the nutrients in the food to keep things running smoothly, while giving us that energy we need to get through our day. When you eat junk food, you are getting the calories, but not the nutrients. As a result, you are likely to eat again soon after, and not burn off the calories in the meantime.

This wouldn't be such a bad thing, except for the fact our bodies store all of those extra calories that are not burned, as fat. That is why people become overweight. Now, you are probably wondering where I am going with all of this.

Let's go back to yoga, and I will show you how all of this ties together. Close your eyes like you did at the beginning of this book, and I want you to imagine a football enthusiast on the day of the super bowl.

Think of what they are wearing, what they are saying, and what they are eating. If you are thinking like the standard answer, you probably said things like pizza, buffalo wings, chips, and beer or soda.

Odds are you are right. Our brains associate those foods with that person. We don't need to know a single thing about them, not their name, their likes or dislikes, their job, or anything, all we needed to know was that they were a football enthusiast, and we were able to say what they were eating.

Now, I want you to picture a person that is a yoga enthusiast. Same drill. What are the wearing? What are they saying? What are they eating? Odds are you imagined a person wearing the standard yoga outfit, someone who is nice, and someone who likes to eat healthy foods.

Probably organics, with a lot of granola, nuts, and berries. Things like that. Of course there are probably some variations in your own mind, but this is the most common answer to that question.

To bring this back to what we were talking about before, think of it this way. When a person becomes a yoga enthusiast, they become free thinkers. They are people who feel closer to nature, and closer to the earth around them.

As a result, they don't want to put things into their bodies that are harmful to them. They naturally start to shift their preferences from McDonald's to places that offer a lot healthier alternatives, and many of them prefer to cook from scratch.

Not that there is anything wrong with McDonald's food in moderation, but this is a major reason why people have problems with their weight. Not that food chain, but fast food in general. Processing food so much is not good for it, and it is not good for us to put in our bodies.

When you embrace this kind of lifestyle, you are going to be amazed at how quickly you want to change what you put into your body, and how your taste will genuinely change for things that are healthier.

Granted, you likely won't be transformed from French fries to spinach overnight, but you will find that those things that are deep fried or heavily processed just don't have the same effect that they once did, and you will begin to prefer the way you feel when you eat things that are better for you.

It becomes a cycle that you will greatly enjoy. You will want to stick with your exercise regime and eat better because you feel better, and you will feel better because you are eating better and sticking with your regime.

When this happens you will start to see a real transformation in your body, which is exciting for anyone, and you will be amazed at how on top of the world you feel. It will be as though nothing can bring you down from your happiness, and you will want to share the feeling with everyone you come into contact with.

In addition to the way you will start to look and feel, you will realize how fun it is to eat right. To go out and find the things that you like, and be able to take them home and prepare them yourself, or to go out and be with other people who feel the same way you do, and want to make themselves better, too.

There really is a fellowship to eating right, and you will be pleasantly surprised at how many people there are who want to swap recipes and make things with you. Who knows, if you are outgoing and confident in your new lifestyle, you may make a likeminded friend who can share the journey with you.

No one likes to walk alone, and I promise you there are a lot of people out there with this mindset. You don't have to look very hard and you will find them, and you will feel so good knowing that you have your own little group of supporters and friends that you can get to know and grow with.

Relaxing With Yoga

While yoga for weight loss is one of the biggest reasons people do it, there are a lot of other benefits from practicing this lifestyle besides on the scale benefits. Call them side effects if you will, because no matter what you are doing yoga for, you are still going to see these things happen in your life as a result.

Don't worry, they are all good and desirable things, and you will be happy to have them. That is one of the beauties of this practice, no matter why you are doing it, you are going to see the benefits come pouring in to your life.

For example, if you are doing yoga to lose weight, you will find that you gain confidence and feel more relaxed. Stress will melt away and your worries will fade. These are all things that come from one who is able to focus on the task at hand, and able to see the finer things in life.

A person who is a yoga enthusiast, and is doing yoga for easing stress and relaxation, will also find that their body is getting in better shape, and that they feel more flexible when they are out and about.

The strain will be gone from their backs and necks as they sit for hours at their desks, and they will sleep better at night, and likely be happier with what the scale says.

If you do yoga because you want to be more flexible, you will again find the stress is eased out of your life and you feel more relaxed. There really is no way to get around the benefits that come from practicing this lifestyle regularly.

Now, you may be wondering how one goes about practicing yoga for relaxation. It isn't as black and white as it is for weight loss, and there are other things you need to factor in before you will see the results.

First, let's take a look at the methods themselves, and figure out how you can use them to relax and ease your stress.

You need to look at the stationary poses. The ones that do not require you to do a lot of balancing, or the ones that cause parts of your body to burn as you work. These are all great for weight loss, but that is not your goal this time.

Focus on the meditation poses, and the poses that are specifically designed to increase flexibility. These are the ones that are going to ease your stress because these are the ones that are meant for well-being.

The first and foremost thing you can do when you are relaxing, is to close your eyes and breathe. Let it out, and clear your mind. Some say to think, but that isn't what you want to do right now. You can think through your problems later. Right now you need to focus on… nothing.

Clear your mind and breathe. To add to this experience, and make it that much more stress free, try timing your meditation. There are guided meditations and timed meditations all over the internet that you can listen to for free.

Say you only want to spend 10 minutes relaxing and meditating? No problem. Simply go to YouTube and search for 10 minute meditation music playlists. There will be so many that you can choose from, and they are all just 10 minutes long.

Once you have decided on which one, spread out your mat and assume a meditation pose. Play the music and simply stay still, breathing your yoga breath and clearing your mind.

It may not seem like much at first, but if you do this every day, you will notice within 3 days how much calmer you feel overall. You will be at peace with this relaxed feeling that just gives a new light to the day.

It really doesn't take a lot of time out of your day, and you will be amazed at how things that used to bother you just don't anymore. All of those things that seemed like such a big deal at the office now seem to be manageable and in line. All because you learned the art of meditation, and there is so much relaxation to be found there you won't have to worry ever again.

The second thing we are going to look at is along the same lines of the act of yoga, but it is in the mind. One who practices yoga is one who is focused. This is an art that will add so much relaxation to your day, you won't believe it.

This is because a person who is focused sees what needs to be done, and does it. They do not worry about what will happen, or what could happen, no, they are only worried about what they can do and what they will do.

A focused person knows there is no point to worrying about things you have no control over. Those are just distractions that are designed to keep you from achieving what it is you have set out to achieve.

If you want to be more relaxed, and use yoga to do it, you need to learn how to be a focused person during the day, and learn how to set time aside for that meditation session.

It really will become and invaluable time to you, and you won't want to miss even one day of doing it. Then again another benefit to yoga is that you know even if you miss a day that it will be ok, and that you will be able to pick up where you left off later.

That is the whole point to using this lifestyle to relax. You gain a perspective that not a lot of people are open to learning, and you will become a person that they are envious of.

Who doesn't want to be relaxed, and self-assured? You are going to be that person that everyone envies, wondering how they, too, can achieve that level of calm and collected.

The Art of Letting Go

A person who practices yoga often is one that is often called 'calm' and 'gentle'. These are true of those that practice, but why are they that way? It isn't as though stretching in different positions a few times a week will make you be a forgiving person.

Or will it?

Maybe not the stretching part, but the mindset does it for them. This is because a person who is in this lifestyle, is a person that feels connected. As you learn more about it, you will see that we are all connected to each other, and that we need to work together on a lot of things, but we will discuss more on that later.

What we are getting at right now, is a person who wants peace, and one who knows the value of connection, is not a person who is going to hold a grudge. They don't have time to.

They know that life is short, and that it is precious. Who has time to hang on to hurt when there is a beautiful world out there? Now I do admit this is all much easier said than done, but hear me out.

A person who thinks through all of this, can see that if they are hanging on to hurt and unforgiveness is ultimately just hurting themselves. There is no one out there on this planet that has the power to make you feel anything.

Your feelings come from within, and you are choosing subconsciously what you feel. Don't believe me? Take this for example. If you are in the grocery store, and you are hit from behind with a cart, you are likely to feel a mix of surprise and anger.

You whirl around, and there is the man who was once that bully all throughout school. He laughs at you and walks away. Now, you are really angry, hurt, and can't wait to tell everyone what has happened to you, that is if you don't act on all of this anger and pick a fight.

Now rewind a little bit. You're back in the store, and you are hit from behind with a cart. Those feelings of surprise and anger well up within you, and you whirl around.

What you see is a little old lady, her cane over her arm, and giant rimmed glasses over her eyes. She apologizes that she is slow, or that she bumped you, and your anger is gone.

In fact, you may feel a bit of humor… over the same act.

Between these two situations, nothing changed for you. You were hit from behind both times and both times you had the same reaction. In the first scenario, you were made fun of, and you 'chose' to hold on to that anger.

In the second, you let it go… but I am about to tell you a secret, you could let it go in *both* situations, regardless of what the other person did or who they were. Going back to the bully. They can do the same thing to you.

Right down to that laugh and walking away, but you are left with a choice. You can now stew over it, feel angry, and feel as though you have been wronged, or you can laugh that there are such petty people out there and move on with your day.

Nothing at all changed for you, but your outlook on the situation changed, and I promise you that you will feel a lot better about yourself if you are driving home, having forgotten the incident entirely, than if you are going home, stewing the whole way about how unjust this world is.

No one has the power to make that choice for you, it is entirely your own. If you are a person that is involved with yoga, you will learn that there is so much good in this life that needs to be pulled to the surface, and you will realize that there isn't time to worry about what the bullies are doing in this world.

And not just the bullies, this needs to apply in every situation you find yourself in. Whether you are dealing with your family, friends, difficult people, easy to get along with people, and everyone in between.

If you want to know what it is like to have true peace, you need to learn how to let it go and move on. There is nothing that has happened to you, or ever could happen to you that could warrant stealing your happiness forever.

Don't get me wrong, there is a lot of bad things that happens in this world, and it happens to good people who do not deserve it, but there is nothing that can happen in this world that will steal your happiness unless you let it.

Of course you are still going to have bad days, and you are still going to be sad from time to time, but you have to learn how to deal with those things in a healthy and timely manner. Don't pout for days over something that went wrong.

Learn where you could have done better, and move on. It never does anyone any good to sit and pout over something, and I promise you that you are the only one whose day is being ruined.

Learn to see the positive in life, and you will find that things are a lot easier to let go of, in fact, the positive nature that you will develop will prove to be contagious, and you will see that there really isn't that much to be sad about.

Life is a good, wonderful, and mysterious gift of untold beauty. You only have one shot to live it, so don't ever waste even a single minute of it.

Joining the Energy

Most people who have heard about yoga are familiar with the concept that there is an energy that surrounds it, waiting to welcome in whoever wants to be a part of it.

Over the course of time, there has been a lot of discussion as to what that energy is, and whether or not it is a real thing, and it is a discussion I am not going to worry about.

You may have already noticed in life, and if you have not yet noticed it you soon will after I point it out, is the fact that people love to be offended, and people love to argue. The more a person can disagree in life, the more they are going to do it, and if they can be offended on top of it, well, that is just the icing on the cake.

Energy in the universe has become one of those topics, and it is something that people will argue about for as long as they can. It really doesn't matter what anyone has to say about it, or what your own personal belief is about it, it is a topic I don't see the need to get into, so I am not going to.

Why? Because getting into that kind of topic or debate is really just splitting hairs, and it is something that one could easily categorize in the let it go chapter that we just looked at. When it comes to the source of the energy you are looking for, do what makes you happy.

No matter how you look at it, the energy is coming from within, and that is what I want to focus on. Mostly because you are the one you have control over, and you are the one who is growing in this lifestyle.

This is a topic with no right answer, and no wrong answer. You need to sort out what you personally believe, and make the most of the energy that comes from that belief. In the meantime, you need to draw on the energy that is in your own soul.

There are things that you need to realize when you are in this kind of life, and that is there are a lot of people who are going to disagree with you. Of course, this is true of any lifestyle simply because people like to argue, but the yoga lifestyle is no exception.

So what do you do? You join the energy, of course.

What makes this such a powerful lifestyle is that you are either in or you are out. There is no middle ground in this, and you are welcome to make your choice as you see fit.

I don't encourage you to try to find a yoga energy to tap into, I encourage you to engage in that energy that is already inside of you. The real you that has been fighting to get out all of this time, but that you have been afraid to let out for fear of what people will think.

The energy that you need to be a part of is the one that free thinkers embrace. The thinking that they know who they are and they want to be who they want to be.

This is the energy you need to tap into. The energy of the free thinkers. Be a person who is a standout in society. Not a person who is an outcast, don't go out of the way to break the rules or be controversial, but also don't be afraid to be yourself.

Remember you are a wonderful and beautiful person just as you are, and you never need to be afraid to express yourself. The more you are yourself, the better you will feel about yourself, and the better you feel about yourself, the happier you will be all around.

Everyone has an energy inside of them, and you do, too. You need to let this out and embrace it for all that it is worth. Never let anyone tell you that you are not good enough, or that you are different for any reason.

There is nothing wrong with being yourself. You will find that we live in a world that tells you to love yourself, but that most people will get mad at you if you do. It is as though they prefer you to be in an unhappy place, because this is where they are comfortable with you being.

Then again, you may find that you are comfortable being there yourself. We get ourselves trapped in these comfort zones whether we like them or not, and we find that we can't break out of them no matter how miserable we are, and this is not healthy.

To be successful in your yoga lifestyle, you need to be able to break free of this sort of thinking, and be willing to push yourself outside of your comfort zone and pursue things that you never thought you would.

The more you push yourself out of your comfort zone, the more comfortable you will feel the next time you need to do it. Comfort zones are things that we do so often that we become comfortable doing them (hence the title) but living in your comfort zone isn't going to take you anywhere in life.

You need to be willing to stand alone, and feed off of your own energy. There is enough positivity inside of you that will last you a lifetime, and you honestly don't need to have another person's approval to be happy in life.

This is one of the most freeing feeling that you will ever achieve in your life. As soon as you let go of the need to have other people's approval, and hang on to the fact you can sustain yourself, you will be able to make your own way in life and not have to feed off of what other people are doing.

More than Movement

Yoga is a movement in more ways than one. First, it is an actual physical movement that you do for a variety of reasons, and secondly, it is a cultural movement.

There are so many people who practice yoga these days, it has become a culture in itself, and it is waiting for you to become a part of it. If this is a lifestyle that you are passionate about, and one that you want to live in, then you need to pursue it like a passion.

There is no need to be shy when it comes to something you are passionate about, and your new lifestyle is no exception. Keep in mind when you decide to join this kind of lifestyle, it is something that is so much more than movement.

Sure, you will find that you are frequently doing a variety of stretches and poses that you will only get better at as time goes by, but there is more to it than that. We have already looked at how doing this often will result in you feeling better, caring more about others and less about your problems, and how you are grasping that energy that is within you.

What all of this is adds up to is the fact that this is a belief in addition to a practice. It is a life that will affect every part of your day, from the moment you get up to the moment you go to bed, and it will have an effect on everything you do in your day.

You will find that you will be a lot less negative, and that you will want to be with people who are positive. Complaining is something that will start to annoy you, and you will be that person who can see some good in everything and everyone.

You will find that there is a new appreciation for the small things in life, both living and material. There is a charm that lies in something as little as a flower growing by the sidewalk, and you will see that there is a majesty to the great buildings we have built.

There is a stunning beauty to the way manmade things and nature collide and coincide, and you will take it all in for what feels like the first time. Yoga has a way of slowing you down, making you reflect and consider what you want in life, and what life has to offer you.

That man that is in the grocery store that grabs the annoying cart... the one you wonder if he is deaf... well, you are going to be that person who enjoys the squeak of a cart for what it is.

There is the realization out there that there is so much in life to be appreciated and cared about, and these are things that are often overlooked and underappreciated.

We have all heard the saying that tells us to slow down and smell the roses that grow along the path, but there is a lot of truth to that statement. Your hundred years on this planet is going to rush by faster than you thought it would, and you will one day be that older person in the nursing home and thinking about the life that you lived.

Some find this to be a sad thought, but it is really a gift to you and to others. In the natural life that you lived, you learned things you will be able to pass on to the next generation. In a world that is being taken over by technology, there are few people out there that really think about the little things in life.

Of course the thought of all of that is leaping ahead of where you are now by decades, but it is something you need to keep in mind right now. Live your life of movement as more than a movement.

Embrace life for its simplicity, and for all that it has to offer. There are enough worries in life to fill your day without you needing to bring in more with fears of things that may or may not happen, and you need to learn to live with these fears for what they are... fears.

A fear in and of itself is not something that can hurt you. You need to realize this and move on from it, whatever that fear may be. Live your life in confidence that it will be ok, no matter what turn your life takes, you are going to make it through.

Hold your head high wherever you go, and whatever situation you are in, and will go far. There is nothing that can stand in between you and your success in life, besides you.

Don't be your own biggest enemy, and don't get weighed down by the things in this life that scare you. That isn't what this movement is about. It is about living life for all that it has to offer, and for everything you can get out of it.

You only have one shot at this whole thing, so don't waste it in any way. There are those that waste it being reckless, and there are those that waste it being paranoid. Your life was not something that happened by chance, and you are hear for a specific purpose.

What you need to do is find out what that purpose is, and live the best life you can with that purpose in mind. Are you meant to be a revolutionary? Are you the one who is going to give this world the wakeup call that it needs?

You very well could be that person, and you need to be ready to rise to that occasion when it arises. Live life as though you are a part of the greatest movement this planet has to offer.

Rise to the challenges, and celebrate the victories, you have one life to live, so make the most of it!

Mind and Body

Yoga and the yoga mindset are two things in one. Just like the mind and the body. Two things that are separate, function separately, yet come together as one. There is nothing more beautiful than two things that are flowing together in perfect sync, and you need to strike this balance in your own life.

With everything we have learned about yoga so far, it may seem to be rather daunting to think of it as something you can mold into perfect sync with itself and you.

The natural life, the organic mindset... these are things that seem to go hand in hand, and they do... until we put them inside a real live person. It is no secret that most people greatly enjoy desserts, fast food, and other unhealthy things.

Of course this is nothing too surprising. Who doesn't' like to have an ice cream cone or a cheese burger? These are a common part of our daily lives, especially if you are one of the busy people that does not have time to carefully plan all of your meals.

What I am driving at here is that you should not get stuck in a stereotype. Yes, you are part of a yoga lifestyle, and yes, you are part of a movement, but you are still you, and that means you still have your own personal tastes and preferences.

Don't get caught in the mindset that you have to do things you don't want to do to be good at yoga, or that there was a way you failed for eating something that wasn't healthy, or that you skipped a few days in the studio.

There is a balance between mind and body that you need to find. Find that spot where you are happy with who you are and what you are doing, but don't let yourself slip into unhealthy habits.

What I mean by this is that there is always a compromise. If you want to have a cheeseburger, for example, go out and get one. Get the cheeseburger that would be considered the worst thing for you by a nutritionist's standards, and enjoy it.

Eat it guilt free and move on. It is your choice, and you are free to be you. Just because you are part of a lifestyle doesn't meant that you can't have things like that, but what you need to avoid is doing that often.

If you want to do it, limit it to once a week. This is a point that goes for whatever the given situation may be. Whether you like to have a drink every now and then, or if your guilty pleasure happens to be candy or chocolate.

Total deprivation is the worst thing you can ever to do yourself. This is because you are only setting yourself up to fail. It isn't a pessimistic outlook to admit you are human, and that there are things you like to have.

As a general rule of thumb, you can have anything you want, you just have to moderate it, and you can't beat yourself up over it later. This is the perfect sync I am talking about when it comes to mind and body.

So many people... especially women... who do this feel guilty that they had something that wasn't necessarily on their 'diet', so they feel that they must then punish themselves by not having anything that they like for a period of time, or that they must then work out for hours on end to burn it off.

A life of beauty and balance is not a life that would ever require you to do that, and that is what I am talking about when I mean that the mind and body are in sync. On the flip side of this topic, you need to listen to your body when your mind is feeling ambitious.

For example, if you know that you haven't worked out for a few days, and you really want to run through a few sequences, but your body is not feeling up to it, don't force yourself to do it. This is a life of balance, and sometimes that means you have to set aside something that you want to do, even if it is something that is good for you... to do something that is better for you.

Be careful that you do not become so firm over the little things that you end up missing the big picture. This life of nature and yoga is supposed to be one of happiness and peace, not one of stress and anxiety. If there is ever anything you are doing that causes you to be stressed out, stop it immediately and move onto something else.

As we were talking about earlier, you have only been given one life to live, and it is far too precious to be wasted on stress and worry. If you are embracing this lifestyle the way it was intended to be lived, you won't ever have reason to stress.

Whenever you find yourself in doubt of a choice you have made, or if you feel guilty that you did something you shouldn't have, stop and take a breath. Just breathe whenever you feel lost or like you need to clear your mind. That is the entire purpose of this life, to make you feel connected enough with yourself and the people around you that you can stop and breathe if you ever need to.

And don't worry if this is something that takes time for you to get used to. We have been talking for a while now that this is a process, and that you have to work towards it, so don't ever get caught up thinking that since you have not gotten there yet, or that since you have some things to work on, that you are a failure, or that you can't do it.

This is a life that was meant to be lived to the fullest, so what are you waiting for? Get out there and take this world for what it is, and the people in it for who they are. Don't worry if it takes time, or if they are worried about you at first.

As much as we would like it to be, this is not a world full of happiness and sunshine. There are going to be those people that you meet that are just a drag, and there are going to be good days and bad days.

I can't promise you that you will never run into a tragedy, or that bad things will never happen to you, no matter what kind of life you live. What I want to do is encourage you that there is a good time and there is a bad time, and that life itself hinges on balance, you just need to learn to focus on that balance.

There are many people who believe there is a lot of appeal in being an extremist, and for them that may be their path, but don't let anyone ever get on you for not being one, too. You know that there is benefit to living a life of balance, and no matter what the rest of the world does, you are going to live your life the way you see fit.

You are a one of a kind human, and there is no one else out there who can be like you, so of course there are going to be people who need time to warm up to you and your way of life, but give them their time, and you take yours.

What is important is that you are happy, and that you are doing the things you care about. Once you have come to this life of balance, you are ready for anything. There is nothing that can phase you, and nothing that can drag you down, because you know that you will be able to make it through, and there will be good times again.

Focus in Motion

The whole key to yoga and being successful at it is mastering the ability to balance. As we looked at in the previous chapter, that means a balance in life as well as in the exercises themselves.

There are many different things you can do to help you improve your balance. Look at a piece of string, or some other object. No matter what happens, while you are doing the pose, look at this object and do not look away.

You will find that if you keep doing this, it will become a lot easier to do the pose. Here is another example. If you try that old balance an egg on your head trick, and you just can't seem to get the egg to stay in place, pick another object that is exactly eye level with you, and watch it no matter what while you have the egg on your head.

Suddenly, having an egg on your head is no big deal, just as you could do that pose. The same rule holds true in nature. As you see a gazelle running from a cheetah, or a cat after a bird... no matter what happens, they do not take their eyes off of their goal, even for a second.

So what do all of these things have in common, and why are we looking at them here?

The answer is simple: These are all great pictures of focus.

In the first two examples, you found that by focusing on a single object while you were doing something else, you were able to accomplish your goal with ease, and in the last two, the animals that were hunting never lost focus, and they were able to catch their prey.

But what does all of this have to do with yoga, and the Namaste lifestyle?

For starters, this is a great way to help you get through those exercises. If you are having a tough time with a pose, focus. Dig deep and look at what you need to get through the exercise.

With practice, you will eventually be able to do it without the object to focus. Not that there is a problem with looking at something while you are trying to pose, but it will help you to learn these poses in a way your body remembers how to do them as a second nature.

But that is all in the physical realm of the benefits of focus, as we know, there is so much more to yoga than stretches, so let's take a look at how focus is an important aspect to have when you are living the yoga lifestyle.

We all know that person. The one who shows up at every party, is always looking to have a good time, is always working some odd job or a small job that is easy to get and hard to lose, but there is something about them that tells you they are not going anywhere in life.

I am not trying to be mean, but I know you understand what I am saying, they seem like a lot of fun, but when it comes down to it, they don't appear to be doing much. Now, to be clear, there really isn't a thing inherently wrong with a person who does this, but it is not a desirable way to be.

It doesn't matter who this person is, how well you know them, what they look like, or how nice they are, they don't have focus in their life.

Focus is the little voice inside of you that keeps you on track with something. Whether it be a new job, or a project, or a long term goal that you have, if you lose your focus, whatever it is you are doing is sure to suffer as well.

But if you stay focused, it doesn't take long at all before you have reached your goal, and are able to set new, harder goals to accomplish. Focus is something that is hard to learn, so you are definitely having a head start if you have the ability to focus.

If you don't, don't be upset. There are different exercises you can do online that will help to improve your focus, and things such as memory games or other things that deal with the mind will help a lot, too. It is a trait that can be acquired if you don't lose interest and stay on topic.

Once you are able to incorporate focus into your day, you will find that there are many new doors opening up to you. Decide which one is the best one to take before you enter, and you will be well on your way to living the life you want to live, and achieving the goals you want to achieve.

Living the Yoga Lifestyle

We have broken down so many different aspects of this lifestyle, I could easily wrap up this chapter in a few lines telling you to now combine all that you have learned, and don't forget to do your exercising.

No yoga book on the planet would be complete if we didn't talk about our carbon footprints. We are all here on this same planet, making the most out of our limited resources. Don't be a person who is careless or selfish with the things that we have been given.

Just as there have been thousands here before us, there are going to be thousands more here after us, and our planet is wearing out. Let's all make an effort to do what we can to make sure the print we leave behind us is small, and that we are not causing pollution in the mean time,

I could say that was all you need to know now, I have covered so many things about this lifestyle you are sure to have your work cut out for you. That wouldn't do much good though, as there are a few more things I would like to share with you.

Above everything else that we have looked over in this book, as you are on your journey to living a life of natural beauty and yoga bliss, you need to remember to lighten up.

Yoga was created for you to enjoy, not for you to become a slave to. You want to make a good impression to the people around you, you don't want to be that person they think is rude, or be that person everyone assumes is arrogant.

This is a lifestyle that says we are all going to make it, and that you want to see other people succeed. There is nothing worse to deal with than jealousy, and that goes for both people involved.

No matter who is around you, or who else you meet, you are incredible, and you know that your greatness comes from within. Just because that other person you know is good at what they do, or if they are successful, or good looking, or anything you can think of, that doesn't make you any less.

Comparison is something that is manmade, and it is ugly. With your yoga life, learn not to compare people to people, or yourself to others. There are too many ways for that to go wrong, and for you to start feeling badly about yourself.

This is a beautiful planet that we live on, and we are supposed to take care of it. Do your part to take care of your own garbage, and the garbage that you see on the street. Never be afraid to work hard, and certainly never be afraid to be the hardest worker in a room.

Take care of others, and be gracious enough to let other people take care of you. This is a journey that we are all in together, and there is no hero. If you want to help people, help them as much as you can, but also know that there are people out there who want to help you, and you need to be able to get them do things for you, to keep their own mind at peace.

Smile often, and let the world know you are happy to be there, and that you are happy that they are there, too. Be kind to everyone, including the animals. They are sweet creatures, and they do their best on this planet as well, so live in harmony.

Forget the things people have done to hurt you, and don't do things that are going to hurt someone else. Don't start arguments, and never back down from what you believe in.

Promote love as often as you can. Don't base it off of anything. What they do, how they dress, who they are, these are all irrelevant things in the big picture. Love is love, and it is something everyone yearns for, and everyone deserves to get.

Make sure you eat right most of the time, and don't freak out about the times that you don't. Workout regularly, but love your body and yourself for who you are. There is no one else on this planet that is better than you. Remember that.

Focus on your goals, both those that are happening now and those that are happening later. Never assume what you do now won't matter later, it always will.

Above all, be happy. All of these things are important, but the end goal is happiness. There is so much joy to be found in the simple things, so live them up while you can, and don't sweat the bad times.

Your world awaits, get out there and live it up for all that it is worth.

**** PREVIEW OTHER BOOKS BY THIS AUTHOR****

"BUDDHISM FOR BEGINNERS" by Dominique Atkinson

[Excerpt from the first 3 Chapters – for complete book, please purchase on Amazon.com]

Chapter 1: Introduction

Buddhism is considered one of the first organized religions arising in the 4th and 5th centuries. With a following of approximately 300 million people around the world, Buddhism was founded approximately 2,500 years ago by Siddhartha Gotama, known more commonly as Buddha. Though it is generally considered to be a religion, Buddhism is more accurately a way of life, leading its followers to be moral, mindful and full of wisdom and understanding. In doing this, followers of Buddhism aspire to attain enlightenment and live a truly fulfilled life.

Buddhist's are constantly surrounded by statues of Buddha. These images are used to remind all followers of the level of peace and happiness that they can achieve through enlightenment. Though followers may appear to worship these idols, what they do is actually pay their respects to a man who become more than just a man; someone who they believe is the true key to their enlightenment.

Although many viewing Buddhism from the outside believe he was God, returned to Earth, this is not the case. He never claimed to be God and instead believed himself to be merely a man who was capable of achieving enlightenment. He was determined to help anyone and everyone (no matter what their background or demographics) achieve enlightenment.

One of the best things about this philosophy or lifestyle is that it is tolerant of all others. Under Buddhism other religions and belief systems are not only tolerated, but accepted and believed in. It actually believes in the teaching of all religions and does not seek to convert those who are presently following other religions. Instead, it only seeks to explain Buddhism to those who are interested in learning it, leaving all others to their own devices, beliefs and religions.

These beliefs definitely make Buddhism very different from most other religions which have spent time, energy and even money in converting others to their beliefs and ideals. There have never been wars or battles fought in the name of Buddhism because acceptance, tolerance and love are taught so strongly as basic tenants of the religion.

Chapter 2: The History of Buddhism

Buddha was born in Nepal in the 6th century B.C. Siddhartha was born to a tribal king. His mother passed away only shortly after his birth. He was shut away in a beautiful palace with only servants to keep him company. Though he was married at the age of 16, he continued to live in seclusion for 13 more years.

The myth is that when he was finally allowed to leave the palace in a chariot, he was amazed and surprised to see so many examples of humanity that had before been kept from him. The first thing he came across was a very old man, to which his chariot driver explained that everyone grew old. Upon another trip outside he came across a diseased man, to which his driver explained, people would grow ill throughout life. A subsequent visit introduced him to a decaying corpse, introducing the understanding that people would someday die. Finally, he was introduced to an ascetic, someone who had given up all worldly things and, simultaneously, fear of death.

He was 29 by this time and decided that he would become an ascetic as well. Leaving behind his beautiful palace and his family, he began to wander the world, seeking a way to relieve suffering. Over a period of six years he amassed a group of five followers and practiced a variety of religions with different teachers. Though he studied and meditated in many forms, he was unable to find the true answer to his quest. It was then he determined to follow a more severe path, fasting entirely without food or water and enduring intense amount of pain at the same time. He was certain that this must be the way to full enlightenment and understanding.

After some time, he determined that this also was not the answer he sought and accepted a bowl of rice from a young girl he met during his travels. Upon eating and drinking as well as finally bathing in the river he determined that there had to be another way to achieve enlightenment than to pursue self-punishment. Though his followers deserted him, Siddhartha determined that there must be no extremism if one was to accomplish the goals he had for himself. The path he then forged, one of balance between pleasure and suffering, was named the 'Middle Way' and is still the way of Buddhists to this day.

Siddhartha determined that he would meditate instead and that, before he rose again, the answer would come to him. It took several days of deep meditation, of looking inside himself, of clearing his mind, of reviewing his life and his past lives, before he found the beautiful state of enlightenment that he had sought. Fighting away the demons which attempted to claim his perfect state, he began to truly see and experience that which he had sought. He could finally understand suffering and had reached enlightenment for himself. It was in that moment he became Buddha.

His first sermon was over 100 miles away, where he found the five individuals with whom he had traveled previously. Though he had initially been uncertain about preaching at all, his first sermon, Setting in Motion the Wheel of the Dharma, allowed him to draw in followers who also wanted to reach the level of enlightenment that he was able to achieve. He outlined to them the Four Noble Truths and the Eightfold Path which will be discussed throughout later sections of this book and his followers created a community of monks known as Sangha to also seek the higher truth that Buddha had achieved. There were no barriers for those who wished to join Sangha and all, despite their race, class, sex or background, were allowed to join in the search for fulfillment.

Buddha continued to preach his sermons and his path to enlightenment until his passing at the age of 80. He became a beacon of hope for many, leading them down the path to fulfillment in their lives and to peace and happiness as well. Through his teachings, known as the Dharma, he was able to draw many more to Buddhism, throughout his own country and beyond as his teachings began to morph throughout the world.

Chapter 3: The Teachings of Buddhism

Throughout his life and his own enlightenment Buddha came to recognize Three Universal Truths, Four Noble Truths and the Noble Eightfold Path. Each of these can be used together to help anyone interested in improving their life. In this chapter we will talk about each of them and throughout the next chapters we'll help you understand more about how to apply each of them specifically to different aspects of your own life.

The Three Universal Truths

Nothing is Lost in the Universe

Buddha came to understand that everything that exists in the universe, from the smallest insect to the largest elephant is there for a purpose. Each creature, each plant is precious to the existence of life as we know it. When a tree dies it decomposes into soil that is used by new trees. When that tree grows it produces the oxygen necessary for life. Because of oxygen, humans are capable of life. This basic tenant led to an understanding of the Buddha and his followers to never kill an animal.

Everything Changes

Life continues to grow. Throughout existence everything in life will continue to change and adapt. And not only does life continue to evolve but it is sometimes positive and sometimes negative. As things continue to advance and change life will never cease. As evidenced by the death and extinction of the dinosaurs, and the continuation of life to the present day, nothing ever truly ends and life will continue to go on.

Law of Cause and Effect

Finally, the Buddha determined that changes will continue to occur because of cause and effect. This idea is considered as karma and it states that everything will occur in a way that is representative of our own actions. When someone commits an action they are at risk of a reaction to occur as well. Though these reactions may be positive (as by someone committing a positive action) they may also be negative. Karma encourages those who follow Buddhism to continue to behave in a positive way at all times.

The Four Noble Truths
Suffering is Common to All

The Buddha emphasizes that suffering will occur and that it is impossible to avoid suffering entirely. As a result, it is important to understand what suffering is. In many situations such as sickness, old age, death or even birth anyone will feel suffering. In other situations however, such as being away from someone that they like and not getting the things that they want in life, many people will go through a period of suffering. And Buddha emphasized that suffering will occur and happiness cannot last forever.

We Are the Cause of Our Suffering

Because so many people live in ignorance and greed they do not live their lives in a way that can improve their karma. They end up with a large amount of bad karma and end up experiencing a lot more suffering. Because they act in a way that is not appropriate, always wanting more, they are incapable of ever achieving true peace and nirvana. This can come from being spoiled and from reaching too much for additional possessions rather than being happy with what one has.

Stop Doing What Causes Suffering

In order to cease the suffering that you are going through you need to give up greed and ignorance (the worst aspects of suffering). For a Buddhist the cessation of these emotions and feelings is called Nirvana. Achieving nirvana will allow for joy and everlasting peace but it is only possible if you are able to stop allowing greed to envelop your life and you are capable of divesting yourself of all desires as well.

Everyone Can Be Enlightened

Finally, anyone can achieve enlightenment. All it takes is following the Middle Way, the Noble Eightfold Path. If you follow this path and you continue to observe all of its teachings you will be capable of living an enlightened life in the same way as the Buddha was able to do. For all of his followers this path was the true way to achieve everything that they have been able to achieve and it is believed to be the best way for anyone else to achieve these same accomplishments as well. Following this path will end suffering.

The Noble Eightfold Path
Right View

In order to achieve spiritual enlightenment and to truly achieve everything that is capable of making you stronger and more fulfilled you must seek to view the world in the proper way. This requires you to look at the world with wisdom and compassion which is the way of the Buddha.

Right Thought

Thinking in a positive and clear way is essential to being able to achieve enlightenment. The Buddha teaches that we are the things that we think and therefore it is crucial that we think properly. By thinking kindly we are able to develop our character properly.

Right Speech

Speaking in the best way possible, speaking in a positive, kind and helpful manner, is the best way to gain the admiration of others. Though admiration is not necessary for full achievement of enlightenment, traits that go along with it such as respect and trust most definitely are.

Right Conduct

To achieve enlightenment it is also imperative that we carry ourselves in an appropriate way. This requires us to behave in the way that is best for the world and not just the way that is best for ourselves. We must also make sure to act in the way that we require others to act.

Right Livelihood

Working is a difficult aspect of Buddhism and of life in general. Because we must all find a way to make a living, it is crucial that we continue to uphold the teachings of Buddha even in our work. According to the Buddha we must do our best to achieve a living through a method that does not bring harm to anyone or anything or cause others to feel unhappy.

Right Effort

In doing the best that we possibly can at all times it is possible achieve much more. This means putting all of our effort forth to achieve what we should be working towards. It means not spending time in ways that are harmful and instead, spending our time in doing our very best in everything that we attempt or accomplish.

Right Mindfulness

Before we think, speak or do anything it is important that we keep in our minds the proper ways of thinking and acting. We must be careful to consider all thoughts and actions before they are committed as, once done, these things are not simple to undo.

Right Concentration

Focus is crucial to success in any endeavor and most especially in this because it allows for the best ability possible to be put forward. Anyone who strives to complete a task must likewise strive to do it well.

In order to use each of these in the best way possible, anyone striving to follow Buddhism and achieve enlightenment must likewise consider the Three Jewels; the three different aspects of Buddhism which will allow them to follow the true path. These Three Jewels are extremely important and include The Buddha himself as the guide to the path, the Dharma (also the Eightfold Path) as the path to follow, and the Sangha as the teachers to lead you on your way.

The Five Precepts

Also included in Buddhism, much in the way they are included in Christianity, are five precepts or 'rules' not to break. Created directly by the Buddha, these instructions for life are crucial to anyone who wishes to achieve enlightenment because breaking them will cause the path to become muddied and potentially impassable as well. This makes it important to understand each aspect and why each aspect is so important to the following of the Buddha and his path.

Do Not Kill

The Buddhist teachings state that to kill one creature (any type of creature) is to bring about the death of oneself. A true Buddhist must have a love and caring for all creatures and must wish them to be free from any type of harm at all times. This goes for any creature from the soil to insects all the way to the largest creatures known to mankind. As such, Buddhists are generally expected to be vegetarian, so as to avoid injuring or killing any animals for their own pleasure or wellbeing.

Do Not Steal

Taking from someone else is showing a disregard for that other person. We must instead seek to provide for others rather than taking from them. In order to provide for others properly we must be sure not to take from them but to give whatever we can and whatever we believe we are able. This involves sharing what is available on our table no matter who with.

Do Not Commit Sexual Misconduct

Buddha believed that behaving in a proper way was the best way to show respect for our own body as well as for our parents who gave us life and the presence of that body. By behaving in a pure and virtuous way it is possible to improve the world in which we live and likewise to improve our own family and our own livelihood at the same time. This requires showing respect for all we come into contact with as well as ourselves.

Do Not Lie

To lie is to take away from the self and from those around you as well. By being honest, avoiding gossip and avoiding idle or harsh speech, it is possible for the world to fall into peace. By talking it is also possible to avoid misunderstanding and to therefore avoid anger.

Do Not Use Intoxicants

Intoxicating substances will only dull the mind and the senses. They will cause quarrel with family and friends and they further cause illness and weakness. As a result, the Buddha believes that there is no place for any type of intoxicants within his teachings. Instead, the body should remain healthy and pure and the mind must be kept clear so it is possible to achieve not only happiness but cleanliness as well. This will provide for enlightenment and for an easier way down the path toward that true enlightenment that the Buddha has promised......

[Excerpt from the first 3 Chapters – for complete book, please purchase on Amazon.com]

www.ingramcontent.com/pod-product-compliance
Lightning Source LLC
Chambersburg PA
CBHW081537280526
45788CB00010B/3266